Dedicated to

_____

The section in the back of this book designated
ACKNOWLEDGMENTS is hereby made
a part of this copyright page.

Illustrations by Kate Greenaway with permission of
Frederick Warne (Publishers) Ltd. London

What Is A Baby?

With the art of
KATE GREENAWAY

Selected by Barbara Shook Hazen

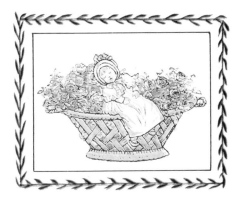

The C.R. Gibson Company, Norwalk, Connecticut

A baby is wonderful...

wonderful,
wonderful,
and most wonderful wonderful!
and yet again wonderful
and after that,
out of all hooping!

Shakespeare

Every child born into the world is a new thought of God, an ever-fresh and radiant possibility.

Kate Douglas Wiggin

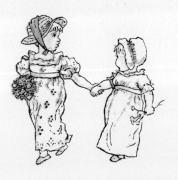

...and full of wonder

How like an Angel came I down!
  How bright were all things here!
When first among His works I did appear
  O how their Glory me did crown!
The world resembled His ETERNITY.
  In which my soul did walk;
And every thing that I did see
  Did with me talk.

Thomas Traherne

God one morning, glad of heaven,
  Laughed—and that was you!

Brian Hooker

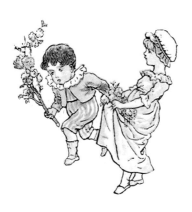

A baby is a brand-new beginning...

Babies are such a nice way to start people.

Don Herold

His first smile, an ear-to-ear effort that reveals his smooth gums and narrows his eyes to half-moons of joy, results in such an exuberant response from me that tears of surprise follow. His first laugh, a chuckle bubbling up at the end of a 3 A.M. feeding, leaves me longing for the next midnight wail. His first poem, "Aah-goo, bah-aah!" lengthens into a ramble through the vowel sounds, and I become his echo.

Claudia S. Brinson

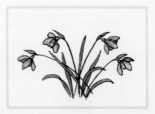

...and a magnificent re-creation

Grandma's eyes,
and Grandpa's grin,
Daddy's ears,
and Mother's skin,
and great Aunt Ann's
dimpled chin
are all come full
circle in him.

Barbara Shook Hazen

Unwritten history
Unfathomed mystery!

Josiah G. Holand

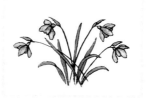

A baby is charming...

TWO DEEP CLEAR EYES

Two deep clear eyes,
Two ears, a mouth, a nose,
Ten supple fingers,
And ten nimble toes,
Two hands, two feet, two arms, two legs,
And a heart through which love's blessing flows.

Walter de La Mare

Bits of star-dust blown from the hand of God.

Larry Barretto

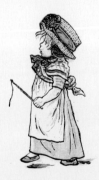

...but a baby is demanding

Ounce for ounce, a baby has more appeal than can be resisted by any adult. Babies are fresh... wholesome...charming...BUT DANGEROUS! They will use their powers every day to get what they want—other kids' toys, endless attention, your valuable stereo equipment, and anything delicate and fragile. It is only with the utmost concentration that new parents can keep any control over their lives at all!

Arlene Stewart and Joan Van Raalte Quill

Because a baby is...
   A perfect example of minority rule.

Milwaukee Journal

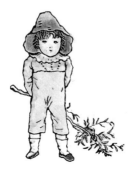

A baby is to rock...

SONG FOR A FIFTH CHILD

Mother, oh mother, come shake out your
　　cloth!
Empty the dustpan, poison the moth,
Hang out the washing and butter the bread,
Sew on a button and make up a bed.
Where is the mother whose house is so
　　shocking?
She's up in the nursery, blissfully rocking!

Oh, I've grown as shiftless as Little Boy Blue
(Lullaby, rockaby, lullaby loo).
Dishes are waiting and bills are past due
(Pat-a-cake, darling, and peek, peekaboo).
The shopping's not done and there's nothing
　　for stew
And out in the yard there's a hullabaloo
But I'm playing Kanga and this is my Roo.
Look! Aren't her eyes the most wonderful hue?
(Lullaby, rockaby, lullaby loo).

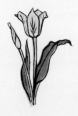

Oh, cleaning and scrubbing will wait till
    tomorrow,
But children grow up, as I've learned to my
    sorrow.
So quiet down, cobwebs. Dust go to sleep.
I'm rocking my baby. Babies don't keep.

Ruth Hulburt Hamilton

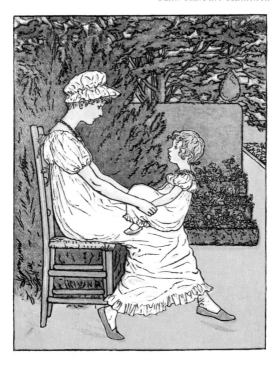

A baby is someone to care for...

Don't take too seriously all that the neighbors say. Don't be overawed by what the experts say. Don't be afraid to trust your own common sense. Bringing up your child won't be a complicated job if you take it easy, trust your own instincts and follow the directions that your doctor gives you. We know for a fact that the natural loving care that kindly parents give their children is a hundred times more valuable than their knowing how to pin a diaper on just right or how to make a formula expertly.

Dr. Benjamin Spock

A baby is a thing on mother's milk and kisses fed.

Homer

...and a big step forward
for the parents

Parenthood is a big step forward that requires a great deal of reconsidering of the past. In the process of learning to be a mother, a woman re-experiences what happened to her when she was being mothered. As she cares for her child, she may feel satisfied that she is taking good care of the child and develop into an even more capable person...Just as the infant gains confidence and self-esteem through a good mother-child relationship, so does the mother.

The Group for the Advancement of Psychiatry

God sends children for another purpose than merely to keep up the race – to enlarge our hearts; and to make us unselfish and full of kindly sympathies and affections; to give our souls higher aims; to call out all our faculties to extended enterprise and exertion; and to bring round our firesides bright faces, happy smiles, and loving, tender hearts.

Mary Howitt

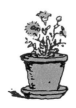

A baby is to hug…

KISSING KIN

I'll get me a pocket
To carry you in
And a filigree locket
The size of your chin,
My dilly, my docket,
My kissing kin.

My pride now has grown
As immense as the nation,
And warm to the bone
Is my new inclination:
Content to be known
As your kissing relation.

Oh, fair is the sight
Of the light of your grin,
And silver-spoon bright
Beams the small soul within,
But love charms against night
Are your kisses, sweet kin.

Elizabeth McFarland

...but is an occasional bother to a brother

BROTHER

I had a little brother
And I brought him to my mother
And I said I want another
Little brother for a change.

But she said don't be a bother
So I took him to my father
And I said this little bother
Of a brother's very strange.

But he said one little brother
Is exactly like another
And every little brother
Misbehaves a bit he said.

So I took the little bother
From my mother and my father
And I put the little bother
Of a brother back to bed.

Mary Anne Hoberman

A baby is a unique
one-of-a-kind individual...

Every single child who is born is different
from every other child. Each of us is only
himself and nobody else.

Eda LeShan

As long as I live
I shall always be
My Self—and no other,
Just me.

Walter de La Mare

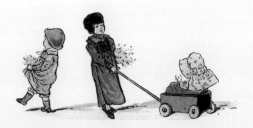

...and today's explorer

From the moment of birth your baby begins to explore his world, first with his eyes and then with his hands. When he can turn over and crawl, he goes after what he sees.

Joseph Sparling and Isabelle Lewis

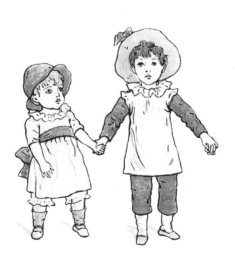

A baby is perpetual motion...

Hop away, skip away
My baby wants to play,
My baby wants to play every day.

Felix Summerly

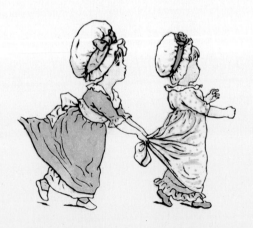

LULLABY, OH, LULLABY!

Lullaby, oh, lullaby!
Flowers are closed and lambs are sleeping;
Lullaby, oh, lullaby!
Stars are up, the moon is peeping;
Lullaby, oh, lullaby!
While the birds are silence keeping,
Lullaby, oh, lullaby!
Sleep, my baby, fall a-sleeping,
Lullaby, oh, lullaby!

Christina G. Rossetti

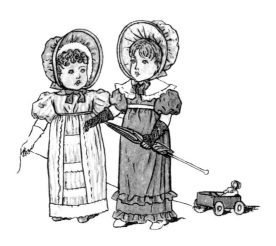

A baby is a gift from God...

BABY

Where did you come from, baby dear?
  Out of the everywhere into the here.

Where did you get those eyes so blue?
  Out of the sky as I came through.

What makes the light in them sparkle and spin?
  Some of the starry spikes left in.

Where did you get that little tear?
  I found it waiting when I got here.

What makes your forehead so smooth and high?
  A soft hand stroked it as I went by.

What makes your cheek like a warm white rose?
  I saw something better than anyone knows.

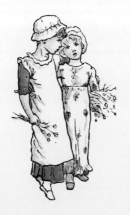
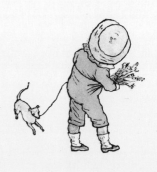

Whence that three-cornered smile of bliss?
  Three angels gave me at once a kiss.

Where did you get this pearly ear?
  God spoke, and it came out to hear.

Where did you get those arms and hands?
  Love made itself into bonds and bands.

Feet, whence did you come, you darling things?
  From the same box as the cherubs' wings.

How did they all just come to be you?
  God thought about me, and so I grew.

But how did you come to us, you dear?
  God thought about you, and so I am here.

George Macdonald

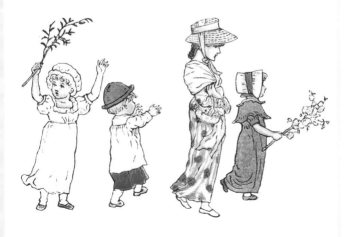

But most of all a baby is to love...

BABY LOUISE

I'm in love with you, Baby Louise!
With your silken hair, and your soft blue eyes,
And the dreamy wisdom that in them lies,
And the faint, sweet smile you brought from the
    skies,–
God's sunshine, Baby Louise,

When you fold your hands, Baby Louise
Your hands, like a fairy's, so tiny and fair,
With a pretty, innocent, saint-like air,
Are you trying to think of some angel-taught
    prayer
You learned above, Baby Louise?

M.E.

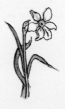

...and love some more

Love is the parent gone wild
With joy by the smile of a child.

Lillian Everts

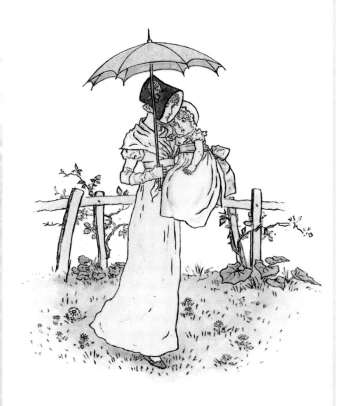

ACKNOWLEDGEMENTS

The editor and the publisher have made every effort to trace the ownership of all copyrighted material and to secure permission from copyright holders of such material. In the event of any question arising as to the use of any such material, the editor and the publisher, while expressing regret for inadvertent error, will be pleased to make the necessary corrections in future printings. Thanks are due to the following publishers and authors for permission to use the material indicated.

BRINSON, CLAUDIA SMITH, for "The Joys of Motherhood." Copyright © by Claudia S. Brinson.

COOPER SQUARE PUBLISHERS, New York, New York for "Wonder" from *The Poetical Works of Thomas Traherne,* ed. Gladys I Wade. Copyright © 1965 by Cooper Square Publishers. p.5.

THE CROWN PUBLISHING GROUP, for "Baby Louise" by M.E. from *Library of World Poetry,* ed. by William Cullen Bryant.

GROUP FOR THE ADVANCEMENT OF PSYCHIATRY, for an excerpt from *The Joys and Sorrows of Parenthood.* Copyright © 1973 by the Group for the Advancement of Psychiatry. Reprinted with the permission of Charles Scribners Sons, publishers.

HAMILTON, RUTH HULBURT, for "Song For A Fifth Child." Copyright © 1958 by Ruth Hulburt Hamilton. Reprinted courtesy of *Ladies' Home Journal.*

HOBERMAN, MARY ANN, for "Brother" from *Hello And Goodby.* Copyright © 1959 by Mary Ann Hoberman. Published by Little, Brown and Company. Reprinted by permission of Russell and Volkening, Inc., agents for the author.

HOFFMAN, ELIZABETH MCFARLAND, for "Kissing Kin" from *The Ladies' Home Journal,* Nov. 1954. Copyright ©1954 by Elizabeth McFarland. Reprinted with permission of the author and *The Ladies' Home Journal.*

HOLT, RINEHART AND WINSTON, PUBLISHERS, for an excerpt from *The Indiscreet Years* by Larry Barretto. Copyright © 1931 by Larry Barretto. Reprinted by permission of Holt, Rinehart and Winston.

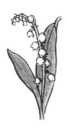

Book design by Bonnie Weber

Type set in Caslon 540 and Caslon 540 Italic